W9-DCC-158

ARTERIOSCLEROSIS
and
HERBAL CHELATION

by
Hanna Kroeger
Minister of the "Chapel of Miracles"

ISBN 1-883713-03-X
© 1984
by
Hanna Kroeger Publications
800-225-8787

DECONGEST YOUR ARTERIES

Over a quarter million aortocoronary bypass surgeries are performed in the United States every year. It is the most frequently performed major surgery in this country. Between 2 and 5 percent of aortocoronary bypass patients have complications from surgeries, including death. Many people who undergo this surgery never fully recover and are unable to return to work. This type of operation relieves the symptoms of heart disease but does not affect the causes.

"It is a sad fact that a surgical intervention constitutes an admission of failure of medical treatment. The surge of aortocoronary bypass operations gives testimony to the absence of effective medical treatment directed to alleviate or eliminate the cause underlying the disease process." *Nutrition News*, December 1982.

ARTERIOSCLEROSIS AND ATHEROSCLEROSIS

"My people are dying from lack of knowledge." These words from the Bible come to me as I write about how arteriosclerosis can be healed.

Arteriosclerosis is a term applied to a pathological condition in which there is thickening, hardening and loss of elasticity of the walls of blood vessels, especially the arteries; in short, it is hardening of the arteries.

Atherosclerosis takes place when arteries are blocked and the blood cannot pass through freely.

Long before it comes to a stroke and/or heart attack, the buildup in the arteries is there. It builds up over the years and arteriosclerosis is no longer a disease specific to senior citizens. Young men in their 30's or even younger show signs of trouble. Recently, researchers found arterial changes in infants. Even women, who were thought to have immunity to arteriosclerosis, suffer more and more from this disease.

When physicians speak about arteriosclerosis, they compare this disease with the plague of the Middle Ages. The question is why are so many people plagued with the buildup of plaque in the arteries? Arteriosclerosis and atherosclerosis are two sides of the same coin. The first one is hardening of the elastic tube, the artery, and filling up these tubes with sludge and blood corpuscles. Atherosclerosis is the fat deposits in and around the arteries, choking the passage of blood and bringing on complete stoppage. The final result of both is a heart attack or a stroke.

HERBAL CHELATION

Herbs, vitamins, minerals and amino acids are a godsend for our health. We can help ourselves by using these important supplements to attain excellent health. They can do wonders for the heart and circulation.

Doctors in Germany recommend hawthorn for people with heart disease. They have learned and applied what herbalists have known for hundreds of years—that hawthorn helps the heart. It is wonderful for problems associated with atherosclerosis, high blood pressure and elevated cholesterol levels. Hawthorn also strengthens heart contractions, lowering blood pressure and lowering pulse rate.

Equisetum arvense is the fancy term for horsetail, which one French medical journal described as having healing properties for the heart. *Equisetum* contains elemental silicon, which is necessary for maintaining flexible arterial walls. As we get older we have less and less silicon and must take *Equisetum* to make up for this loss. When *Equisetum* is combined with hawthorn, the results are amazing. *Equisetum* acts like a broom for the arteries and increases the number of blood corpuscles.

People with heart disease lack chromium and selenium. Our food used to supply us with these minerals but now the soil is losing precious nutrients due to over farming and harsh chemical fertilizers. Animals who graze on selenium depleted soils have weakened heart muscles. Chromium is very important because it improves the ratio of "good" cholesterol to "bad" cholesterol and keeps the overall cholesterol level down. We should consider supplementing with these minerals to avoid complications.

Amino acids can be remarkable for the heart, especially taurine and arginine. Taurine is known to benefit with hardening of the arteries, high blood pressure and even congestive heart failure. This amino acid protects against potassium depletion of the heart, which can lead to seriously irregular heartbeats. Taurine is needed to maintain proper blood platelet functioning. The amino acid arginine is the only source for nitric oxide, which is vital for healthy blood vessels in order to relax the arterial walls so that blood can flow more freely.

Vitamin C helps with blood clotting and high cholesterol levels. It also maintains capillary wall strength. Vitamin C and selenium are important antioxidants for those with heart conditions to protect against stroke.

These items are so divine that they have been referred to as Our Lord's Formula. Aloe vera gel is also recommended to keep circulation flowing.

Take *Herbal Chelation* with 2 tbsp. aloe vera gel before each meal 3 times daily. You can take aloe vera gel alone or put it in apple juice or water but *not* in citrus juices.

Do this for 1 month and then have your physician recheck the health of your arteries. If it is not all gone, repeat. Do not eat heavy meals, potato chips, heavy cakes, alcohol or strong coffee.

In order to keep arteries clear afterwards, consider the French method: 1 kelp tablet and 1 choline tablet (250 mg) 2 times daily.

Yogurt and applesauce is a specific to keep arteries clean.

Reports

"I was scheduled for bypass operation. I knew that only 1 to 4 percent of people die on the operation table, so I was not worried about that and, yet, the closer the scheduled date came, the more nervous I became.

"A friend of mine suggested the cleaning out of the arteries with Our Lord's Formula. First I said, 'Impossible,' but I had nothing to lose, so I started taking Our Lord's Formula with aloe vera gel 3 times daily and also at bedtime. One week went by. I felt better. I could take a deeper breath. I could sleep better. Another week went by and I had no more pressure in my chest. Then I postponed the operation for 2 weeks and after 4 weeks I saw my doctor again. We both could not believe it. The arteries around the heart where they wanted to make the bypass were clear."

Walter Brown, IA

"The pain in my legs was killing me. I could hardly walk 1 or 2 blocks, then I had to rest from pain. My arteries were clogged in the lower extremities. That's what I was told. I went on the Lord's Formula. After only 2 days I found relief. I kept on taking it for 4 weeks and I can walk all I want to without pain."

A. Solari, Denver, CO

"I lost my memory. I could not think of the past or keep my daytimes straight. 'Old age,' my daughter said. I misplaced the car keys, I could not remember the TV show, I could not think any longer. A pounding headache came, announcing the inevitable stroke. My daughter found a lady who had taken the Lord's Formula and she brought one month's supply to try it. The month passed. I can think again. First the pounding left. Then my eyes got better and now I can think. I will always treasure this recipe."

Irene Burger

"I had had two chelation therapies and soon needed a third one. I found Our Lord's Formula amazing. I tried it. It worked like a charm. No more trouble."

Eric Warding

"My bypass operation was successful, however, after a year, claudication set in. I limped at times. I had leg pains. I felt tired, exhausted, sleepless. At times my eyes blurred and I was scared. The Lord's Formula worked. No more trouble and it is so easy. No side effects, no pain and no economical disaster—$25 took care of it."

Hilde Bishop, Fort Collins, CO

"My asthma left me after using the Formula for one month."

Anne Myer

SYMPTOMS OF ARTERIOSCLEROSIS

What symptoms does your body give you when plaque is building up in the arteries?

- Watch for an overly tired feeling after a heavy meal.
- Observe forgetfulness with tasks that you normally perform with acuity.
- Notice if your mind will not grasp new ideas or follow new dimensions.
- Persistent feeling of weakness, coldness, tingling or burning in your toes or feet.
- Be aware of dull headaches.
- Persistent sleeplessness is another danger signal.
- Tightness in chest.
- Pain in shoulders when not accident related.
- Breathlessness when walking or lifting.
- Notice if walking gives you pain in the calves of the legs and that, when you rest, you feel better and pain will disappear.
- Notice if you had a good night's sleep. You get up and stretch or exer-

cise. In the middle of the sternum is a sharp pain. It will go away and not return until the next morning when the same pain returns at the same time in the middle of the sternum.
- Notice if there are small ulcerations of your skin on ankles or feet.
- Notice head noises, dizziness, sudden spells of partial deafness.
- Notice blurred or darkened vision.

SYMPTOMS OF ADVANCED ARTERIOSCLEROSIS

The first signs of plaque buildup in the arteries are not easily recognized. We talked about this already. Symptoms of advanced arteriosclerosis are when the stricken person makes very small steps and has to rest every 100 to 200 yards because of pain in feet and/or legs, particularly calves. Sometimes they limp (it is called claudication) but this is always accompanied with pain. This could be arteriosclerosis in the lower extremities.

Symptoms that may have an underlying cause of blockage in the arteries (a plaque buildup in arteries so that blood and oxygen are not sufficiently supplied to the different organs of the body) are:

• Asthma	• Leg pain
• Heart trouble	• Lymph trouble
• High blood pressure	• Liver trouble
• Loss of memory	• Kidney trouble
• Loss of sleep	• Diabetes
• Loss of hearing	• Prostate trouble
• Loss of eyesight	• Stroke

It sounds harsh, but there is no better prevention and correction of the above disease patterns than the cleaning of your arteries.

When diseased, the venous system can also make pain and give trouble similar to arterial blockage. Here is the difference to observe: When you walk briskly and tightness and pain start in calves and feet and will let up when you stand for a little while, that shows an arterial blockage. In a venous system blockage, pain diminishes as you walk but, when you stand still, pain increases.

7

WHAT CAUSES ARTERIOSCLEROSIS
AND ATHEROSCLEROSIS?

This is what experts tell us:

• Too much fat intake.
• Too many chemicals in food, water and air.
• Too many metals in food, water and air.
• Too much sodium fluoride buildup.
• Too much sugar (more than 6 tsp. at one time causes blood to coagulate, making tiny blood clots).
• Too much environmental stress.
• Too little exercise.
• Too much smoking.
• Birth control pills.
• Noise pollution is a definite cause of arterial changes.

Kurt Oster, M.D. added that milk cannot be utilized totally unless it is soured, as in yogurt or kefir. His Xanthine Oxidase theory sounds promising. Read Dr. Oster's book. Also read *Fluoride: The Aging Factor* by Dr. John Yiamouyiannis. A fine work of knowledge is presented here.

In 1945, a hospital in Milwaukee designed for mentally disturbed senior citizens was supervised by E. Seiler, M.D., psychiatrist. She ordered all milk removed from the diet. Only yogurt was permitted once a day. Patients had plenty of butter, oils, vegetables, eggs and meats but no milk or ice cream. The results were astounding. After three months the patients became rational and could be taken home. Many of them kept well for years.

TEST YOUR OWN ARTERIAL HEALTH

Foot Test

Walk barefoot for 2 minutes outside in the grass, if possible. Then lie on your back and stretch your legs upwards. Ask someone to look at the soles of your feet. If they show white spots, it indicates that your leg arteries are narrowed down and not enough blood can reach your feet.

Fist Test
1) Lift both hands above your head.
2) Make fists with firm pressure.

3) Open and close fists 10 times.
4) Ask someone to hold your wrists firmly.
5) Open and close again 10 times.
6) Your helper should release the grip on your wrists quickly. In 4 seconds your hands should be really red. If not, you have arterial trouble in your upper torso.

Eye Test

Look in a mirror. Around the colored part of the eye you will find a white ring.

Ear Test

Look at your ear lobes. A crease in the left ear lobe or a star of wrinkles shows arterial trouble around the heart.

WHERE IS THE BLOCKAGE?

You can find out where the blockage is located.

• Pain around hips and the muscle you sit on becoming lame easily may indicate plaque buildup in aorta.
• Pain in thigh may indicate sclerotic buildup in midsection.
• Pain in calves may indicate arterial trouble in arteries leading to legs.
• Pain in feet and toes may indicate a plaque buildup of arteries supplying blood to the feet.

SENECA INDIAN CLEANSING DIET

The Seneca Indians contributed the following diet:

First Day: Eat only fruits and all you want. Try apples, berries, watermelon, pears, peaches, cherries, whole citrus fruits and so forth, but *no bananas*.

Second Day: Drink all the herbal teas you want, such as raspberry, hyssop, chamomile or peppermint. You may sweeten the tea slightly with honey or maple sugar.

Third Day: Eat all the vegetables you want. Have them raw, steamed or both.

Fourth Day: Make a big pot of vegetable broth by boiling cauliflower, cabbage, onion, green pepper, parsley or whatever you have available. Season with sea salt or vegetable broth cubes. Drink only this rich mineral broth all day long.

This diet has the following effect: The first day the colon is cleansed (your wastebasket). The second day you release toxins, salt and excessive calcium deposits in the muscles, tissues and organs. The third day the digestive tract is supplied with healthful, mineral rich bulk. On the fourth day the blood, lymph and inner organs are mineralized. That makes a lot of sense!

YOU NEED ALOE VERA GEL
FOR CLEANSING YOUR ARTERIES

What is aloe vera? Aloe vera is a plant. It has been used for medicinal purposes for centuries. It has been known for its therapeutic advantages and healing properties for more than 4,000 years. Ancient and modern literature abound with references to this unique, natural remedy. It is sometimes called the medicine, miracle or burn plant.

The Greeks, as early as 333 B.C., identified aloe vera as a medicinal herb. The Chinese considered aloe vera sacred and used it for stomach and colon ailments. In the Philippines it is used with milk for dysentery and kidney infections. The Egyptians used it for sunburns and to retard the aging process.

Aloe vera gel aids in assimilation, circulation and elimination. It has been reported to increase endurance and energy and to provide a speedy recovery from fatigue. It has been known to aid in muscle function and utilization of vitamins and minerals. Aloe vera gel assists in achieving healthy skin and hair.

Aloe vera gel is not a drug. It does not react with medications.

Some properties in aloe vera gel:

Active Ingredients	Minerals	Vitamins
Amino acids	Calcium	A
Enzymes	Magnesium	E
Natal aloes	Sodium	K
Aloin	Potassium	B_1
Emodin	Strontium	B_2
Bitter resins	Boron	B_3
Barbaloin	Silicon	B_6
Chlorophyll	Copper	Folic acid
Albumin	Manganese	Choline
Essential oils	Iron	
Gum arabic	Aluminum	
Silica	Lithium	
Phosphate of zinc	Nickel	
	Zinc	

Other agents of aloe vera gel:

- Pain killer
- Fungicidal
- Germicidal
- Virucidal
- Anti-inflammatory: similar to steroid effects
- Antipyretic: reduces fever and heat of sores
- Natural cleanser
- Penetrates tissue
- Dilates capillaries
- Enhances normal cell proliferation: regenerative stage of healing
- Reduces bleeding time

CHOLESTEROL

As already mentioned, arteriosclerosis and atherosclerosis are two sides of the same coin. With atherosclerosis, a fatty, waxy substance clogs arteries inside and out.

The Greek word *athere* means porridge or gruel and the word athero-sclerosis is the buildup of a gruel-like substance, called cholesterol, in the blood vessels. "The arteries are so plugged up in some autopsy subjects, that no blood can get through at all," commented a first year medical student.

This abnormal condition with its fatal consequences has caused much controversy over the last 10 years and has been called the plague of modern times. It causes 55 percent of all deaths in the United States and has been the leading cause of death in our country since 1920. Scientists estimate that everyone over the age of 21 suffers to some extent from atherosclerosis and/or arteriosclerosis .

Because of the epidemic proportions that this disease has reached, 20 percent of all research monies spent are used to study it and some interesting findings are being disclosed.

Cholesterol is absolutely essential to the body for the production of bile, for fat absorption in the intestines, for steroid hormone synthesis and as an element in cell membranes. Why do we have trouble with cholesterol buildup when the body needs cholesterol? Atherosclerosis is a complex biochemical problem with no simple answers.

The liver is supposed to make the right amount of cholesterol. A poor liver being overworked and maltreated makes short cuts so that the cholesterol amount is larger and more like glue.

The Truth on Cholesterol

Eskimos are on a high fat, high protein diet. They show very high cholesterol but no arteriosclerosis is found. Their arteries are free of cholesterol buildup. Why?

Cholesterol has two chemicals. LDL, which stands for Low Density Lipoprotein, brings the cholesterol from the liver to the tissue. HDL, which stands for High Density Lipoprotein, removes the excess cholesterol from the tissues and arteries. I call it the "Ajax of the arteries." It is arterial cleansing.

Eskimos have lots of HDL; therefore, their arteries are clean in spite of their high consumption of fats and proteins. (By the way, Eskimos have very efficient kidneys to handle all of the protein they consume.)

A Japanese laboratory found that, in the right shinbone, a special hormone is formed which is picked up by the white corpuscles and delivered to the liver to be utilized for cholesterol processing. Since, in some cases, this hormone is at short supply, cholesterol-triglyceride trouble starts.

Here is an herbal formula that helps to create the missing hormone:

- Okra
- Male fern
- Beth root
- Rhubarb root
- Calamus root

A cup of tea made from arnica and hyssop, 3 times daily, is also helpful.

WHAT CAN BE DONE?

- Please quit your smoking. Nicotine constricts arteries and less blood can circulate through the constricted vessels.
- More walking, more foot exercises.
- Garlic is splendid to make arteries soft and pliable.
- B-complex helps a lot.
- Noise pollution weakens the arteries. Workers subjected to loud music or working under motor noises are prone to high blood pressure and arteriosclerosis.
- Avoid too much salt.
- Avoid too much sugar.
- Choline relaxes the arteries and helps in the fibrillation and irregularity of the heartbeat. Choline is easily counteracted by the enzyme cholinesterase; therefore, it has to be taken frequently. Choline is better assimilated in its natural form and you will find an abundance of it in wheat germ, malt and grapes. If you combine choline tablets with kelp tablets, cholinesterase cannot counteract choline so easily.
- Bee pollen is a terrific food supplement, especially in regard to supporting your arteries—$^1/_4$ tsp. 2 times daily will do.
- Folic acid builds the "Ajax of the Arteries," HDL (High Density Lipoprotein).
- In any case, clean out your arteries with *Herbal Chelation and aloe vera gel.*

PROTECT YOUR ARTERIES

It is important for you to keep your arteries clean. What follows is a simple method that comes from England. It is highly recommended to protect your arteries once a year.

First Day: Grind up 1 almond, place in 1 cup of water and drink.

Second Day: Take 2 almonds, place in 1 cup of water and drink.

Third day, etc.: Take 3 almonds and on and on until you have reached 15 almonds.

Then go down step by step until you are back to 1 almond a day. This also is the best remedy I know to prevent cancer.

DECONGEST YOUR BLOOD

Your blood and platelets form an unwanted glue-like substance. If glue-like substances in the blood are allowed to accumulate, the platelets release a dangerous waste called adenosine diphosphate, or ADP. Once ADP is released, other platelets glue together. They form clumps that obstruct the flow of blood through the vessel and this may lead to blood clots in the heart (heart attack), brain (stroke), lung or other vital organs.

Take some onions and cut them into pieces. Add to water and simmer to make onion water. White and red onions together have more anticlotting power.

Drink $\frac{1}{2}$ cup onion water 5 times daily and take 50 mg B_6 with each $\frac{1}{2}$ cup of onion water. Bananas and tomatoes, rice and millet are allowed.

Do this for 2 days in a row. Then pick up a good healthy diet but continue with vitamin B_6. Red clover leaf tea is excellent.

You are as old as your arteries. Old age sets in when arteries are blocked. Old age sets in when parts of your body do not receive enough oxygen or nourishments due to diminished blood supply.

My advice: Clean your arteries with *Herbal Chelation* and aloe vera gel.

Books by Hanna

"Wholistic health represents an attitude toward well being which recognizes that we are not just a collection of mechanical parts, but an integrated system which is physical, mental, social and spiritual."

Ageless Remedies from Mother's Kitchen

You will laugh and be amazed at all that you can do in your own pharmacy, the kitchen. These time tested treasures are in an easy to read, cross-referenced guide. (92 pages) ISBN: 1-883713-04-8

Allergy Baking Recipes

Easy and tasty recipes for cookies, cakes, muffins, pancakes, breads and pie crusts. Includes wheat free recipes, egg and milk free recipes (and combinations thereof) and egg and milk substitutes. (46 pages) ISBN: 1-883713-02-1

Alzheimer's Science and God

This little booklet provides a closer look by presenting Hanna's unique and religious perspectives. (15 pages) ISBN: 1-883713-10-2

Arteriosclerosis and Herbal Chelation

A booklet containing information on Arteriosclerosis causes and symptoms. (14 pages) ISBN: 1-883713-03-X

Cookbook for Electro-Chemical Energies

The opening of this book describes basic principles of healthy eating along with some fascinating facts you may not have heard before. The rest of this book is loaded with delicious, healthy recipes. A great value. (106 pages) ISBN: 1-883713-13-7

Free Your Body of Tumors and Cysts

Hanna brings together many natural techniques, including diet, herbs, vitamins, hands-on healing and more in a practical, understandable approach to growths and their relationships to parasites, cancer and leukemia. (77 pages) ISBN: 1-883713-18-8

God Helps Those Who Help Themselves

This work is a beautifully comprehensive description of the seven basic physical causes of disease. It is wholistic information as we need it now. A truly valuable volume.
(196 pages) ISBN: 1-883713-11-0

Good Health Through Special Diets

This book shows detailed outlines of different diets for different needs. Dr. Reidlin, M.D. said, "The road to health goes through the kitchen not through the drug store," and that's what this book is all about. (90 pages) ISBN: 1-883713-14-5

Hanna's Workshop

A workbook that brings together all of the tools for applying Hanna's testing methods. Designed with 60 templates that enable immediate results.

How to Counteract Environmental Poisons

A wonderful collection of notes and information gleaned from many years of Hanna's teachings. This concise and valuable book discusses many toxic materials in our environment and shows you how to protect yourself from them. It also presents Hanna's insights on how to protect yourself, your family and your community from spiritual dangers.
(53 pages) ISBN: 1-883713-15-3

Instant Herbal Locator

This is the herbal book for the do-it-yourself person. This book is an easy cross-referenced guide listing complaints and the herbs that do the job. Very helpful to have on hand.
(109 pages) ISBN: 1-883713-16-1

Instant Vitamin-Mineral Locator

A handy, comprehensive guide to the nutritive values of vitamins and minerals. Used to determine bodily deficiencies of these essential elements and combinations thereof, and what to do about these deficiencies. According to your symptoms, locate your vitamin and mineral needs. A very helpful guide. (55 pages) ISBN: 1-883713-01-3

New Book on Healing

A useful reference book full of herbal, vitamin, food, homeopathic and massage suggestions for many common health difficulties. This book is up-to-date with Hanna's work on current health issues. (155 pages) ISBN: 1-883713-17-X

New Dimensions in Healing Yourself

The consummate collection of Hanna's teachings. An unequated volume that complements all of her other books as well as her years of teaching.
(150 pages) ISBN: 1-883713-09-9

Old-Time Remedies for Modern Ailments

A collection of natural remedies from Eastern and Western cultures. There are more than 20 fast cleansing methods and many ways to rebuild your health. A health classic.
(105 pages) ISBN: 1-883713-05-6

Parasites: The Enemy Within

A compilation of years of Hanna's studies with parasites. A rare treasure and one of the efforts to expose the truths that face us every day. (62 pages) ISBN: 1-883713-07-2

The Pendulum, the Bible and Your Survival

A guide booklet for learning to use a pendulum. Explains various aspects of energies, vibrations and forces. (24 pages) ISBN: 1-883713-08-0

Spices to the Rescue

This is a great resource for how our culinary spices can enrich our health and offer first aid from our kitchen. Filled with insightful historical references.
(64 pages) ISBN: 1-883713-12-9

Hanna's Books Published by Hay House

Heal Your Life with Home Remedies and Herbs

A compilation of *Ageless Remedies from Mother's Kitchen, Instant Herbal Locator, Instant Vitamin-Mineral Locator, New Book on Healing, New Dimensions in Healing Yourself, Old-Time Remedies for Modern Ailments* and *Spices to the Rescue.*
(296 pages) ISBN 1-56170-512-8

Healing with Herbs A – Z

A compilation of *Ageless Remedies from Mother's Kitchen, Instant Herbal Locator, Instant Vitamin-Mineral Locator, New Book on Healing,* and *Spices to the Rescue.*
(145 pages) ISBN 1-56170-488-1

The Basic Causes of Modern Diseases and How to Remedy Them

A republished version of *God Helps Those Who Help Themselves.*
(162 pages) ISBN 1-56170-527-6